KAPLAN

Related Kaplan Books

MCAT Physical Sciences Flashcards

Get Into Medical School: A Strategic Approach

MCAT Comprehensive Review with CD-ROM

MCAT Practice Tests

MCAT 45

KAPLAN®

MCAT®
Biological Sciences Flashcards

By the Staff of Kaplan, Inc.

Simon & Schuster

NEW YORK · LONDON · SYDNEY · TORONTO

Kaplan Publishing
Published by Simon & Schuster
1230 Avenue of the Americas
New York, NY 10020

Contributing Editor: Albert Chen
Editorial Director: Jennifer Farthing
Project Editor: Anne Kemper
Production Manager: Michael Shevlin
Content Manager: Vanessa Torrado-Caputo
Interior Page Layout: Dave Chipps
Cover Design: Cheung Tai and Mark Weaver

June 2005

10 9 8 7 6 5 4 3 2 1
Manufactured in the United States of America
Published simultaneously in Canada

ISBN 0-7432-7140-8

How to Use This Book

Kaplan's *MCAT® Biological Sciences Flashcards* is perfectly designed to help you learn 350 MCAT Biological Sciences concepts in a quick, easy, and fun way. Simply read the category, Biology or Organic Chemistry, and the item name on the front of the flashcard; then flip to the back to see its definition and subcategory.

The following categories and subcategories have been included in the book, listed in alphabetical order by the two major MCAT Biological Sciences categories and their subcategories.

Biology

- The Cell
- Enzymes
- Cellular Metabolism
- Reproduction
- Embryology
- Musculoskeletal System
- Digestion
- Respiration
- Circulation
- Homeostasis
- Endocrine System
- Nervous System
- Genetics
- Molecular Genetics
- Evolution

Organic Chemistry

- Nomenclature
- Isomers
- Alkanes
- Aromatic Compounds
- Alcohols and Ethers
- Aldehydes and Ketones
- Carboxylic Acids
- Carboxylic Acid Derivatives
- Amines and Nitrogen-Containing Compounds
- Purification and Separation
- Carbohydrates
- Amino Acids, Peptides, and Proteins

Once you've mastered a particular item, clip or fold back the corner of the flashcard so that you can zip right by it on your next pass through the book. The flashcard book is packed with information—remember to flip the book over and flip through the other half!

Looking for still more MCAT prep? Be sure to pick up a copy of Kaplan's *MCAT® Comprehensive Review with CD-ROM*, complete with a full-length practice test.

Good luck!

Biology

ACTIVE TRANSPORT

An amphoteric compound with no net electric charge.

Amino Acids, Peptides, and Proteins

The Cell

Movement of particles from a region of lower concentration to a region of higher concentration utilizing energy.

ZWITTERION

Organic Chemistry

Biology

BACTERIOPHAGES

Amino Acids, Peptides, and Proteins

Three-dimensional structure of a peptide that results from hydrophobic and hydrophilic interactions between residues far apart on the chain. Disulfide bonds and hydrogen bonds can also add to the tertiary structure of the protein.

The Cell

Viruses that can only infect bacteria.

TERTIARY STRUCTURE OF PROTEINS

Organic Chemistry

Biology

CHLOROPLAST

Amino Acids, Peptides, and Proteins

Regularly repeating local structures such as α-helices and β-pleated sheets often formed by hydrogen bonds between residues that are nearby on the chain.

The Cell

The site of photosynthesis in plants. The chloroplast contains chlorophyll, is semiautonomous, and has two cell membranes.

SECONDARY STRUCTURE OF PROTEINS

Organic Chemistry

Biology

CYTOSKELETON

Amino Acids, Peptides, and Proteins

Different polypeptide chains, each referred to as a subunit, associate together to form a functional protein.

The Cell

The cytoskeleton gives the cell mechanical support, maintains shape, and functions in motility. It is composed of microtubules, microfilaments, and intermediate filaments.

QUATERNARY STRUCTURE OF PROTEINS

Organic Chemistry

Biology

FACILITATED DIFFUSION

Amino Acids, Peptides, and Proteins

The sequence of amino acids in a polypeptide, read from the N-terminus to the C-terminus.

The Cell

Passive movement of particles from a region of higher concentration to a region of lower concentration using carrier molecules. Does not require energy.

PRIMARY STRUCTURE OF PROTEINS

Organic Chemistry

Biology

LYSOSOME

Amino Acids, Peptides, and Proteins

The point at which a compound is electrically neutral.

The Cell

Membrane-bound vesicles that contain hydrolytic enzymes used for intracellular digestion.

ISOELECTRIC POINT

Organic Chemistry

Amino Acids, Peptides, and Proteins

Proteins that require a covalently bonded prosthetic group to function properly. Hemoglobin is an example of such a protein.

MITOCHONDRIA

Biology

The site of aerobic respiration that provides the cell with a majority of its energy in the form of ATP. The mitochondrion is a semiautonomous organelle enclosed by two membranes, with an intermembrane space in between the two membranes and a mitochondrial matrix enclosed by the inner membrane.

CONJUGATED PROTEINS

OBLIGATE INTRACELLULAR PARASITES

Carbohydrates

The conversion of an α anomer to a β anomer that occurs when a sugar ring opens, rotates about the bond between C1 and C2, and closes.

The Cell

Organisms that require a host cell to express their genes and reproduce.

MUTAROTATION

Organic Chemistry

Biology

OSMOSIS

Carbohydrates

The smallest unit of carbohydrates. Glucose and fructose are examples of monosaccharides (sugars).

The Cell

Passive movement of water from a region of higher water concentration to a region of lower water concentration; diffusion of water.

MONOSACCHARIDES

Organic Chemistry

Biology

SIMPLE DIFFUSION

Carbohydrates

Sugar that contains a ketone group.

The Cell

Passive movement of particles from a region of higher concentration to a region of lower concentration without the use of energy.

KETOSE

Organic Chemistry

ACTIVATION ENERGY

Carbohydrates

The bond that forms when the hemiacetal group of one sugar reacts with a hydroxyl group on another sugar to form an acetal group in between the two sugars. Polysaccharides are held together by glycosidic linkages.

Enzymes

The difference in potential energy between the initial state (reactants) and the transition state. Reactants must overcome the activation energy in order to undergo the reaction.

GLYCOSIDIC LINKAGE

Organic Chemistry

Biology

ALLOSTERIC ENZYME

Carbohydrates

Isomers that differ in configuration at only one stereogenic center.

Enzymes

An enzyme with two or more active sites that can exist in more than one conformation, usually an active form or an inactive form.

EPIMERS

Organic Chemistry

Carbohydrates

Cyclic stereoisomers that differ in configuration at the hemiacetal carbon (C1). In a six-membered ring, if the hydroxy group attached to C1 and the substituent attached to C5 are trans, the molecule is referred to as the α anomer. If both groups are cis, then the molecule is referred to as the β anomer. Note that C1 and C5 are carbons adjacent to the oxygen in the ring.

APOENZYME

Biology

Enzymes

An enzyme that requires cofactors in order to become catalytically active.

ANOMER

Organic Chemistry

Biology

COMPETITIVE INHIBITOR

Carbohydrates

Sugar that contains an aldehyde group.

Enzymes

Molecule that inhibits the activity of an enzyme by directly binding to the active site of the enzyme. This type of inhibition is usually reversible and can be overcome by increasing the substrate concentration.

ALDOSE

Organic Chemistry

Purification and Separation

A separation technique used to separate a mixture of solids from impurities that have different vapor pressures. The sample is heated under a vacuum. As it sublimes directly into the gaseous phase, the gas is condensed on a cold surface.

ENZYMES

Biology

Enzymes

Protein catalysts that accelerate reactions by reducing the activation energy without being consumed or altered by the reaction. Note that enzymes only affect the rate of reaction and not the amounts of products formed.

SUBLIMINATION

Organic Chemistry

Purification and Separation

Type of chromatography used to separate proteins based on mass. SDS binds to the proteins, giving them a large negative charge canceling the effect of the charges from the individual amino acids. Lighter proteins travel faster than heavier ones.

FREE ENERGY CHANGE

Biology

Enzymes

The difference in potential energy between the initial state (reactants) and the final state (products). A negative ΔG indicates a spontaneous reaction whereas a positive ΔG indicates a nonspontaneous reaction.

SDS-PAGE

Organic Chemistry

Biology

HOLOENZYME

Purification and Separation

A separation technique used to purify the particles of interest from a mixture of solids. The mixture is dissolved in saturating amounts in warm solvent. As the solution cools, the pure substance crystallizes while impurities remain in solution.

Enzymes

An active enzyme containing all necessary cofactors.

RECRYSTALLIZATION

Organic Chemistry

Biology

INDUCED FIT HYPOTHESIS

Purification and Separation

Type of chromatography used to separate proteins based on charge. The stationary gel has an established pH gradient and the proteins (mobile phase) will travel to the point where the pH equals their isoelectric point.

Enzymes

Theory of enzyme catalysis which states that the partial binding of a substrate to an enzyme alters the structure of the enzyme so that its active site becomes complementary to the structure of the substrate, enabling binding.

ISOELECTRIC FOCUSING

Organic Chemistry

LOCK AND KEY THEORY

Purification and Separation

A separation technique used to separate solids from a liquid. This technique utilizes a filter which allows liquids and small particles to pass through while retaining larger particles.

Enzymes

Theory of enzyme catalysis stating that the active site's structure is complementary to the structure of the substrate.

FILTRATION

Organic Chemistry

Biology

MICHAELIS CONSTANT

Purification and Separation

A method used to separate a component in a mixture by exploiting its solubility properties. Usually two solvents are used (one aqueous and one organic) and the component of interest will be soluble in one phase while the impurities will be soluble in the other solvent.

Enzymes

Michaelis constant, K_m, is the ratio of the breakdown of an enzyme-substrate complex to its formation in simple Michaelis-Menton reactions. K_m is also half V_{max}, and a low K_m indicates a strong affinity between an enzyme and its substrate.

EXTRACTION

Organic Chemistry

Biology

NONCOMPETITIVE INHIBITOR

Purification and Separation

A separation technique used to separate liquids with different boiling points. The mixture is heated slowly and as the liquid with the lower boiling point converts into its gaseous form it passes through a condenser where it cools back into its liquid form.

Enzymes

Molecule that inhibits the activity of an enzyme by binding to a regulatory site on the enzyme, thereby changing the conformation of the enzyme. Because these inhibitors do not directly compete with the substrate, increasing substrate concentration usually has little effect on the catalytic rate.

DISTILLATION

Organic Chemistry

Biology

REGULATOR

Purification and Separation

A separation technique that uses the retention time of a compound in the mobile phase as it travels through the stationary phase to separate compounds with different chemical properties.

Enzymes

A molecule, other than the substrate, that can bind to the allosteric site of an enzyme and either increase its activity (allosteric activator) or decrease its activity (allosteric inhibitor).

CHROMATOGRAPHY

Organic Chemistry

Biology

ZYMOGEN

Purification and Separation

A separation technique used to separate particles according to mass, shape, and density. Particles of greater mass and density settle near the bottom of the test tubes while lighter compounds remain on top.

Enzymes

Enzyme that must undergo processing before it can catalyze reactions.

CENTRIFUGATION

Organic Chemistry

Biology

CITRIC ACID CYCLE

Purification and Separation

Type of chromatography that is used to separate nucleic acids based on size. The agarose gel serves as the stationary phase and the nucleic acid serves as the mobile phase. The negatively charged nucleic acids travel toward the anode. Smaller strands of nucleic acids travel faster than larger ones.

Cellular Metabolism

The cycle begins when the two-carbon acetyl group from acetyl CoA combines with oxaloacetate to form citric acid. This product then proceeds through a series of reactions that result in the regeneration of oxaloacetate and the production of 3 NADH, 1 $FADH_2$, and 1 GTP.

AGAROSE GEL ELECTROPHORESIS

Organic Chemistry

Biology

ELECTRON TRANSPORT CHAIN

Amines and Nitrogen-Containing Compounds

An amine where the nitrogen atom is attached to two alkyl chains (HNR_2).

Cellular Metabolism

A chain of cytochromes and other proteins in the inner membrane of the mitochondria that transfers electrons from NADH and $FADH_2$ to oxygen. The energy released from the series of oxidations is used to create a proton gradient which ATP synthase uses to synthesize ATP.

SECONDARY AMINE

Organic Chemistry

Biology

ENERGY CARRIERS (NAD^+, $NADP^+$, FAD)

Amines and Nitrogen-Containing Compounds

An amine where the nitrogen atom is attached to one alkyl chain (H_2NR).

Cellular Metabolism

Molecules involved in cell respiration that serve as energy stores, releasing energy when oxidized to NAD^+, $NADP^+$, and FAD.

PRIMARY AMINE

Organic Chemistry

Biology

FACULTATIVE ANAEROBE

A nitrogen triple bonded to a carbon.

Amines and Nitrogen-Containing Compounds

Cellular Metabolism

An organism that makes ATP by aerobic respiration if oxygen is present but that can switch to fermentation when oxygen is not available.

NITRILE

Organic Chemistry

FATTY ACID ACTIVATION

Amines and Nitrogen-Containing Compounds

An amino group attached to a carbon in a carbon–carbon double bond.

Cellular Metabolism

Fats must be activated using 2 ATP molecules before they can be converted into acetyl CoA and enter the citric acid cycle.

ENAMINES

Organic Chemistry

Biology

FERMENTATION

Carboxylic Acid Derivatives

An alkyl magnesium halide that is used to make carbon–carbon bonds. The alkyl group in a grignard reagent has a negative charge and acts as a nucleophile attacking electrophilic carbons.

Cellular Metabolism

Process by which the cell is able to replenish the NAD^+ used during glycolysis by oxidizing NADH. In this process pyruvate (the product of glycolysis) is reduced by NADH to form ethanol (in yeast) or lactic acid (in humans).

GRIGNARD REAGENT

Organic Chemistry

Biology

GLYCOGEN

Carboxylic Acids

Strong intermolecular bond between a hydrogen atom bonded to an electronegative atom (F, O, or N) and lone electron pairs on either F, O, or N.

Cellular Metabolism

The form in which carbohydrates are primarily stored in the liver. Glycogen is easily converted to glucose-6-phosphate when the body needs it.

HYDROGEN BONDING

Organic Chemistry

Biology

GLYCOLYSIS

Aldehydes and Ketones

Isomers that can interconvert by exchanging the location of a proton.

Cellular Metabolism

Through a series of enzymatic reactions in the cytoplasm, glucose is converted into 2 molecules of pyruvate. The energy released in this process is used to produce a net yield of 2 ATP and 2 NADH molecules.

TAUTOMERS

Organic Chemistry

Biology

OXIDATIVE PHOSPHORYLATION

The process by which the carbonyl oxygen of a ketone gets protonated to form an enol.

Aldehydes and Ketones

Cellular Metabolism

The coupling of the oxidation of NADH, NADPH, and $FADH_2$ with the phosphorylation of ADP. The electron transport chain utilizes oxidative phosphorylation to produce ATP.

ENOLIZATION

Organic Chemistry

Biology

PYRUVATE DECARBOXYLATION

Alcohols and Ethers

Primary alcohols can be oxidized to aldehydes using PCC and further oxidized to carboxylic acids using $KMnO_4$, $Na_2Cr_2O_7$, or CrO_3. Secondary alcohols can be oxidized to ketones using any of the above oxidants.

Cellular Metabolism

The first stage of cellular respiration. Pyruvate is oxidized to acetate, which then combines with coenzyme A to form acetyl CoA in the mitochondrial matrix. This process results in the formation of 1 NADH per pyruvate molecule or 2 NADH per glucose molecule.

OXIDATION OF ALCOHOLS

Organic Chemistry

Biology

SUBSTRATE LEVEL PHOSPHORYLATION

Aromatic Compounds

Describes a situation where the atomic connectivity remains unchanged while the electron distribution between the atoms changes.

Cellular Metabolism

The transfer of a phosphate group from an organic compound to ADP. Glycolysis and the citric acid cycle utilize substrate level phosphorylation to produce ATP.

RESONANCE

Organic Chemistry

Biology

ALLELES

Aromatic Compounds

The term used to describe benzene when it is used as a substituent.

Reproduction

Genes coding for alternative forms of a given trait.

PHENYL

Organic Chemistry

Biology

BINARY FISSION

Aromatic Compounds

The rule stating that in order for a ring to be aromatic it must contain $4n+2$ conjugated pi electrons.

Reproduction

Method of asexual reproduction by which prokaryotes divide. The circular DNA molecule replicates and then moves to opposite sides of the cell. The cell then divides into two daughter cells of equal size.

HUCKEL'S RULE

Organic Chemistry

Aromatic Compounds

Deactivating substituents are electron-withdrawing substituents already attached to the aromatic ring. They decrease the ring's potential to react with other species. With the exception of halogens (which are ortho/para directing) deactivating species are meta directing.

CENTROSOME

Biology

Reproduction

The portion of the cell containing the centrioles.

DEACTIVATING SUBSTITUENTS

Organic Chemistry

Biology

CHROMATIN

Aromatic Compounds

The term used to describe toluene substituted at the methyl position when it is used as a substituent.

Reproduction

Chromosomes in their uncoiled active state. Chromatin is not visible under a light microscope.

BENZYL

Organic Chemistry

Aromatic Compounds

Cyclic, fully conjugated planar compound with $4n+2$ pi electrons. Each atom in the compound must possess a p orbital in order to allow for maximum conjugation.

CORONA RADIATA

Biology

Reproduction

Outer layer of cells surrounding the oocyte. These cells are secreted by follicle cells.

AROMATIC COMPOUND

Organic Chemistry

Aromatic Compounds

Activating substituents are electron-donating substituents already attached to the aromatic ring. They increase the ring's potential to react with other species. Activating species are ortho/para directing.

CROSSING OVER

Biology

Reproduction

The exchange of genetic material between chromosomes (usually homologous chromosomes), that occurs during prophase I of meiosis. Crossing over aids in evolution and genetic diversity by unlinking linked genes.

ACTIVATING SUBSTITUENTS

Organic Chemistry

Alkanes

Bimolecular nucleophilic substitution reactions occur through a concerted mechanism where the nucleophile attacks as the leaving group starts to leave. Reactivity increases from tertiary to secondary to primary with decreasing steric effects.

DIPLOID

Biology

Reproduction

Diploid cells have two copies of each chromosome, usually one from the mother and one from the father. Eukaryotic somatic cells are diploid.

S_N2 REACTIONS

Organic Chemistry

Biology

DISJUNCTION

Alkanes

Unimolecular nucleophilic substitution reaction. Leaving group leaves forming a carbocation which then reacts with a nucleophile. Reactivity increases from methyl to primary to secondary to tertiary with increasing carbocation stability.

Reproduction

The separation of homologous chromosomes during anaphase I of meiosis.

S_N1 REACTION

Organic Chemistry

Biology

DIZYGOTIC TWINS

Alkanes

A carbon atom bonded to two other carbon atoms.

Reproduction

Results when two ova are fertilized by two different sperm. Since the two resulting embryos develop from distinct zygotes they do not have identical alleles.

SECONDARY CARBON

Organic Chemistry

Biology

FOLLICLES

Alkanes

A species that tends to donate electrons to another atom. Nucleophiles are attracted to positive charge. For nucleophiles with the same attacking atom (OH^-, CH_3O^-) in aprotic solvents, nucleophile strength correlates to basicity. In protic solvents and in situations where the attacking atom is different (OH^-, SH^-), nucleophile strength correlates to size.

Reproduction

A multilayered sac of cells that protects and nourishes the developing ovum.

NUCLEOPHILE

Organic Chemistry

Biology

HAPLOID

Alkanes

Atoms that can dissociate to form a stable species after accepting electron pairs. Weak bases tend to be good leaving groups.

Reproduction

Haploid cells have only one copy of each chromosome. Germ cells in humans are haploid.

LEAVING GROUP

Organic Chemistry

Biology

HOMOLOGOUS CHROMOSOMES

Carbon adjacent to the carbon containing the functionality under consideration.

Alkanes

Reproduction

Chromosomes in a diploid cell that contain different alleles for the same trait at corresponding loci.

ALPHA CARBON

Organic Chemistry

Biology

INTERKINESIS

Isomers

Compounds with the same molecular formula but different connectivity. Structural isomers have different chemical and physical properties.

Reproduction

A short rest period between meiosis I and meiosis II during which DNA is not replicated. Ova remain in interkinesis until they are fertilized by a sperm.

STRUCTURAL ISOMERS

Organic Chemistry

Biology

INTERPHASE

Isomers

Compounds with the same molecular formula and connectivity but different arrangement in space. Stereoisomers include geometric isomers, diastereomers, enantiomers, conformational isomers, and meso compounds.

Reproduction

Phase of the cell cycle in which cell division does not take place. Includes the G1 phase, S phase, and G2 phase. Cells in this phase may or may not be growing.

STEREOISOMERS

Organic Chemistry

INTERSTITIAL CELLS

Isomers

A mixture that contains equal amounts of the (+) and (−) enantiomers. Racemic mixtures are not optically active.

Reproduction

Also referred to as "cells of Leydig," interstitial cells are located in the testes and secrete testosterone and other androgens.

RACEMIC MIXTURE

Organic Chemistry

Biology

MEIOSIS

Isomers

A stereoisomer with an internal plane of symmetry. Meso compounds are optically inactive.

Reproduction

A two-phase cell division in germ cells that results in the formation of 4 haploid cells from 1 diploid cell.

MESO COMPOUND

Organic Chemistry

Isomers

Isomers that differ in the arrangement of substituents around a double bond. Geometric isomers are often differentiated using either the cis/trans notation for simple compounds or Z/E notation for more complex compounds, and can differ in their physical and chemical properties.

MITOSIS

Biology

Reproduction

Cell division and/or nuclear division in somatic cells that results in the daughter nucleus receiving a full complement of the organism's genome.

GEOMETRIC ISOMERS

Organic Chemistry

Biology

MONOZYGOTIC TWINS

Isomers

Nonsuperimposable stereoisomers that are mirror images of each other. Enantiomers differ in configuration at every chiral center but share the same chemical and physical properties in a nonstereospecific environment. Optical activity is different.

Reproduction

Results when a zygote splits into two embryos. Since both embryos contain identical alleles, they are often called identical twins.

ENANTIOMERS

Organic Chemistry

Biology

PARTHENOGENESIS

Isomers

Stereoisomers that are not mirror images of each other. Diastereomers differ in their configuration in at least one chiral center and share the same configuration in at least one chiral center. They have the same chemical properties but different physical properties.

Reproduction

The development of an unfertilized egg into an adult organism with haploid cells.

DIASTEREOMERS

Organic Chemistry

Biology

POLAR BODY

Isomers

Stereoisomers that differ by rotation about one or more single bonds, usually represented using Newman projections.

Reproduction

A small, short-lived haploid cell created during oogenesis that receives very little cytoplasm, organelles, and nutrients.

CONFORMATIONAL ISOMER

Organic Chemistry

Biology

PRIMARY SPERMATOCYTES

Isomers

A molecule that is not superimposable upon its mirror image. In order for a molecule to be chiral, it must have at least one chiral center (a central atom attached to four different atoms). However, a molecule with multiple chiral centers can be achiral (meso compound).

Reproduction

Diploid cells that undergo meiosis I to form two haploid secondary spermatocytes.

CHIRAL MOLECULE

Organic Chemistry

Biology

SEMEN

Nomenclature

A compound that has a nonterminal carbonyl group. Ketones are named by replacing the -e in the corresponding alkane with -one.

Reproduction

The fluid discharged during ejaculation. Semen consists of sperm cells and seminal fluid (fluid from the prostate and bulbourethral glands).

KETONE

Organic Chemistry

Biology

SEMINIFEROUS TUBULES

Nomenclature

A compound that has carbon double-bonded to nitrogen.

Reproduction

Located in the testes, the seminiferous tubules are the site of sperm production.

IMINE

Organic Chemistry

Biology

SISTER CHROMATIDS

Nomenclature

Alkanes with a halogen substituent. The compound can either be named as a haloalkane or as an alkyl halide.

Reproduction

After replication each chromosome consists of two identical chromatids held together at a central region called the centromere. After the mitotic spindle pulls the sister chromatids apart, each chromatid is referred to as a chromosome.

HALOALKANES

Organic Chemistry

Biology

SOMATIC CELLS

Nomenclature

A compound that has an oxygen attached to two alkyl groups (R—O—R'). The compound can be named either as an alkoxyalkane or as alkyl ether.

Reproduction

All cells excluding the germ (reproductive) cells.

ETHER

Organic Chemistry

Biology

SPERMATOZOA

Nomenclature

A compound that has a COOR group. Esters are named as alkyl or aryl alkanoates.

Reproduction

Mature sperm specialized for transporting the genetic information from the male to the ovum.

ESTER

Organic Chemistry

Nomenclature

A compound that has an COOH terminal group. Carboxylic acids are named by replacing the -e in the corresponding alkane with -oic acid. Formic acid and acetic acid are common names for the simplest carboxylic acids methanoic acid and ethanoic acid, respectively.

TETRAD

Biology

Reproduction

Four chromatids that result when a pair of homologous chromosomes synapse during prophase I of meiosis.

CARBOXYLIC ACID

Organic Chemistry

Biology

ZONA PELLUCIDA

Nomenclature

A compound in which a carbon atom is bonded to a nitrogen atom with a single bond. Amines are named by replacing the -e in the corresponding alkane with -amine. Substituent groups attached to the nitrogen can be named using the prefix N-.

Reproduction

Inner layer of cells surrounding the oocyte. These cells are secreted by follicle cells. Penetration of the Zona pellucida by a sperm forces the secondary oocyte to undergo meiosis II.

Organic Chemistry

AMINE

Biology

ALLANTOSIS

Nomenclature

A compound that has a carbonyl group bonded to nitrogen. Amides are named by dropping the -oic acid in the corresponding acid and adding -amide. Substituents attached to the nitrogen are listed following N-.

Embryology

The embryonic membrane that contains the growing embryo's waste products.

AMIDE

Organic Chemistry

Biology

AMNION

Nomenclature

Compounds containing carbon–carbon triple bonds. The compound is named by replacing the -ane in the corresponding alkane with -yne.

Embryology

The innermost extraembryonic membrane that contains amniotic fluid in which the growing fetus is suspended.

ALKYNES

Organic Chemistry

Biology

BLASTULATION

Nomenclature

Compounds containing carbon–carbon double bonds. The compound is named by replacing the -ane in the corresponding alkane with -ene.

Embryology

The process by which a morula develops into a blastula with a fluid-filled cavity called a blastocoel.

ALKENES

Organic Chemistry

Nomenclature

Compounds consisting of only carbons and hydrogens bonded with sigma bonds. As chain length increases, boiling point, melting point, and density increase. However, chain branching decreases both boiling point and density.

CHORION

Biology

Embryology

The outermost extraembryonic membrane; contributes to the formation of the placenta.

ALKANES

Organic Chemistry

Biology

DETERMINATE CLEAVAGE

Nomenclature

A compound that has a HC=O as a terminal group. Aldehydes are named by replacing the -e in the corresponding alkane with -al. Formaldehyde, acetaldehyde, and propionaldehyde are common names used for the simplest aldehydes.

Embryology

A cleavage whose future differentiation pathways are determined.

ALDEHYDE

Organic Chemistry

Nomenclature

A compound containing an –OH group. The compound is named by replacing the -e in the corresponding alkane with -ol.

DUCTUS ARTERIOSUS

Biology

Embryology

A shunt that connects the pulmonary artery to the aorta in order to bypass the fetal lung.

ALCOHOL

Organic Chemistry

Biology

DUCTUS VENOSUS

Evolution

Type of natural selection where the normal phenotype is favored while those outside the norm are eliminated.

Embryology

A shunt that connects the umbilical vein to the inferior vena cava in order to bypass the fetal liver.

STABILIZING SELECTION

Biology

Biology

ECTODERM

Evolution

Similar structures that share a common origin.

Embryology

The outermost of the three primary germ layers, which gives rise to the skin and the nervous system.

HOMOLOGOUS STRUCTURES

Biology

Biology

ENDODERM

Evolution

Type of natural selection where both phenotypic extremes are favored over the normal phenotype.

Embryology

The innermost of the three primary germ layers, which gives rise to the linings of the digestive and respiratory tracts, parts of the liver, pancreas, thyroid, and bladder.

DISRUPTIVE SELECTION

Biology

Biology

ENDOMETRIUM

Evolution

Type of natural selection where one extreme phenotype is favored over the normal and other extreme phenotypes.

Embryology

The mucosal lining of the uterus where the embryo implants. Progesterone is necessary for the maintenance of the endrometrium during pregnancy.

DIRECTIONAL SELECTION

Biology

Biology

FORAMEN OVALE

Evolution

Similar structures that share a common function but not similar origins.

Embryology

A shunt that connects the right atrium to the left atrium in order to bypass the fetal lung.

ANALOGOUS STRUCTURES

Biology

GASTRULATION

Molecular Genetics

Class of RNA bearing an anticodon (complementary to the codon) and the amino acid for the corresponding codon. tRNA is vital in translation as it brings the amino acids to the ribosome and insures that each codon matches up with the proper amino acid.

Embryology

The process by which a single-layer blastula becomes a three-layered gastrula.

TRNA (TRANSFER RNA)

Biology

Biology

INDETERMINATE CLEAVAGE

Molecular Genetics

The transfer of information from an RNA molecule to a polypeptide. The three stages of polypeptide synthesis (initiation, elongation, and termination) require energy and are mediated by various enzymes. During translation, mRNA is read in the 5' to 3' direction.

Embryology

A cleavage that results in cells maintaining their totipotency—or ability to develop into a complete organism.

TRANSLATION

Biology

Biology

INDUCTION

Molecular Genetics

A replicated molecule of DNA contains one strand from the original DNA molecule (used as the template) and a newly synthesized DNA strand.

Embryology

The influence of a group of cells sometimes called the organizer on the development of other cells. Induction is achieved by chemical substances known as inducers.

SEMICONSERVATIVE REPLICATION

Biology

Biology

INNER CELL MASS

Molecular Genetics

Class of RNA that is a structural component of ribosomes. rRNA is synthesized in the nucleolus.

Embryology

The group of cells in a blastocyst (mammalian blastula) that develop into the embryo.

RRNA (RIBOSOMAL RNA)

Biology

Biology

MESODERM

Molecular Genetics

RNA is similar to DNA except the sugar in RNA is a ribose and adenine pairs with uracil instead of thymine.

Embryology

Primary germ layer that lies in between the ectoderm and the endoderm. Gives rise to the musculoskeletal system, circulatory system, excretory system, gonads, connective tissue throughout the body, and portions of the digestive and respiratory organs.

RIBONUCLEIC ACID

Biology

Biology

NEURAL CREST CELLS

Molecular Genetics

An enzyme in retroviruses that uses RNA strands as templates for synthesizing cDNA molecules.

Embryology

Cells at the tip of the neural fold; gives rise to many components of the peripheral nervous system.

REVERSE TRANSCRIPTASE

Biology

Biology

PLACENTA

Molecular Genetics

A system that is normally "turned on" but can be inactivated by the addition of a repressor or a corepressor.

Embryology

The organ formed by the uterus and the extraembryonic membranes of the fetus. The placenta contains a network of capillaries through which exchange between the fetal circulation and maternal circulation takes place.

REPRESSIBLE SYSTEM

Biology

Biology

UMBILICAL CORD

Molecular Genetics

Cytosine and thymine are called pyrimidines. They have characteristic monocyclic nitrogenous bases and pair with purines in double-stranded DNA in order to keep the width of the strand constant.

Embryology

Connects the vasculature of the fetus to the placenta.

PYRIMIDINES

Biology

Molecular Genetics

Adenine and guanine are called purines. They have characteristic bicyclic nitrogenous bases and pair with pyrimidines in double-stranded DNA in order to keep the width of the strand constant.

ZYGOTE

Biology

Embryology

A fertilized egg.

PURINES

Biology

Biology

APPENDICULAR SKELETON

Molecular Genetics

A type of RNA polymerase that adds short segments of RNA during replication to which DNA polymerase can add nucleotides. Without primase, DNA replication cannot be initiated.

Musculoskeletal System

The bones of the pelvis, the pectoral girdles, and the limbs.

PRIMASE

Biology

AXIAL SKELETON

Molecular Genetics

In eukaryotes, once an RNA molecule is transcribed it is spliced and a 5' cap as well as a 3' poly-adenine tail are added. RNA in prokaryotes does not undergo such processing.

Musculoskeletal System

The skull, vertebral column, and the bones of the chest.

POST-TRANSCRIPTIONAL RNA PROCESSING

Biology

Biology

CARTILAGE

Molecular Genetics

Mutation in which one nucleotide base is substituted by another. The protein products are usually functional.

Musculoskeletal System

A firm, elastic, translucent connective tissue consisting of collagenous fibers embedded in chondrin. Produced by cells called chondrocytes. Cartilage is the principal component of embryonic skeletons and can harden and calcify into bone.

POINT MUTATION

Biology

Biology

COMPACT BONE

Molecular Genetics

Small fragments of DNA that form the lagging strand.

Musculoskeletal System

Much more dense than spongy bone, compact bone consists of haversian systems (osteons).

OKAZAKI FRAGMENTS

Biology

Biology

FREQUENCY SUMMATION

Molecular Genetics

Class of RNA that is created from the transcription of DNA and serves as the template for protein synthesis during translation.

Musculoskeletal System

The strengthening of contraction that results when the stimuli are so frequent that muscle cannot fully relax. The stronger contraction is due to the incorporation of more muscle fibers.

MRNA (MESSENGER RNA)

Biology

Biology

OSTEOBLASTS

Molecular Genetics

Phase in viral replication in which the host cell is lysed and releases new virons.

Musculoskeletal System

Cells in the bone tissue that secrete the organic constituents of the bone matrix. Osteoblasts develop into osteocytes.

LYTIC CYCLE

Biology

Biology

OSTEOCLASTS

Molecular Genetics

Phase in viral replication when the DNA of the bacteriophage becomes integrated in the host's genome and replicates as the bacteria replicates.

Musculoskeletal System

Cells in the bone matrix that are involved in bone degradation.

LYSOGENIC CYCLE

Biology

Biology

OSTEONS

Molecular Genetics

The strand of DNA that is continuously synthesized in the 5' to 3' direction. The template strand is read in the 3' to 5' direction.

Musculoskeletal System

The structural unit of compact bone that consists of a central canal called the haversian canal surrounded by a number of concentric rings of bony matrix called lamellae.

LEADING STRAND

Biology

Biology

RED FIBERS

Molecular Genetics

The strand of DNA that is synthesized in small fragments called Okazaki fragments and then ligated together. The Okazaki fragments are synthesized in the 5' to 3' direction but the overall synthesis is in the 3' to 5' direction. The template strand has a 5' to 3' polarity.

Musculoskeletal System

Slow-twitch muscle fibers. They are primarily aerobic and contain many mitochondria and myoglobin.

LAGGING STRAND

Biology

Biology

REFRACTORY PERIOD

Molecular Genetics

Segments of noncoding eukaryotic mRNA that are spliced out and not translated.

Musculoskeletal System

A short period of time immediately following an action potential in which neurons or muscle cells are unresponsive to a stimulus. In some cases, a stimulus that is much larger than the threshold causes an action potential in a cell in a refractory period (relative refractory period).

INTRONS

Biology

Molecular Genetics

A system in which a repressor bound to an operator prevents transcription. Addition of inducers can activate an inactive inducible system by preventing the repressor from binding to the operator.

SARCOMERE

Biology

Musculoskeletal System

The structural unit of striated muscle. It is composed of thin (mostly actin) and thick (mostly myosin) filaments.

Biology

SARCOPLASMIC RETICULUM

Molecular Genetics

An enzyme that unwinds the double helix of a DNA molecule, allowing replication to take place.

Musculoskeletal System

A modified form of endoplasmic reticulum, which stores calcium that is used to trigger contraction when the muscle is stimulated.

HELICASE

Biology

Molecular Genetics

Mutation in which a number of nucleotides (except multiples of three) are either deleted or inserted. Such mutations lead to a shift in the DNA reading frame and often result in the translation of nonfunctional proteins.

SPONGY BONE

Biology

Musculoskeletal System

Lighter and less dense than compact bone, it consists of an interconnecting lattice of bony spicules (trabeculae). The cavities between the spicules contain bone marrow.

FRAME SHIFT MUTATION

Biology

Biology

THRESHOLD VALUE

Molecular Genetics

Segments of coding eukaryotic mRNA that are spliced together and translated.

Musculoskeletal System

The minimal value that must be reached in order for the system to respond. Muscle fibers and neurons exhibit an all-or-none response, where the system initiates an action potential only if the threshold value is met.

Biology

TRANSVERSE TUBULES

Molecular Genetics

Plasmids that have the ability to integrate into the host genome.

Musculoskeletal System

A system of tubules that provides channels for ion flow throughout the muscle fibers to facilitate the propagation of an action potential.

Biology

WHITE FIBERS

Molecular Genetics

An enzyme that polymerizes a complementary DNA strand in the 5' to 3' direction using a template DNA strand. A primer is necessary for DNA polymerase to initiate polymerization.

Musculoskeletal System

Fast-twitch muscle fibers. They are primarily anaerobic and fatigue more easily than red fibers.

DNA POLYMERASE

Biology

Biology

BILE

Molecular Genetics

Enzyme that covalently links the Okazaki fragments together.

Digestion

An alkaline fluid synthesized in the liver, stored in the gall bladder, and released into the duodenum. Bile aids in the emulsification, digestion, and absorption of fats.

DNA LIGASE

Biology

Biology

CARDIAC SPHINCTER

Nonoverlapping group of three bases that code for a particular amino acid.

Molecular Genetics

Digestion

A valve between the esophagus and the stomach that prevents the content of the stomach from going back up through the esophagus.

CODON

Biology

Biology

CHEMICAL DIGESTION

Genetics

An allele that is normal to the population.

Digestion

Enzymatic breakdown of large molecules into smaller molecules.

WILD TYPE

Biology

Biology

CHOLECYSTOKININ

Genetics

A form of chromosomal rearrangement in which a portion of one chromosome adds on to a nonhomologous chromosome.

Digestion

CCK is a hormone that is secreted by the duodenum in response to the presence of chyme. CCK stimulates the release of bile and pancreatic enzymes into the small intestine.

TRANSLOCATION

Biology

Biology

CHYME

Genetics

A cross between an organism of an undetermined genotype and another that is homozygous recessive for the trait of interest.

Digestion

Combination of partially digested food and acid that forms in the stomach.

TEST CROSS

Biology

Biology

EPIGLOTTIS

Genetics

The proportion of gametes that receive recombinant chromosomes. If the recombination frequency of two particular traits is high, then it can be inferred that they lie far apart on the same chromosome.

Digestion

A flap of cartilage that covers the glottis when swallowing food in order to prevent food particles from entering the larynx.

RECOMBINATION FREQUENCY

Biology

Biology

GASTRIC GLANDS

Genetics

The physical manifestation of an individual's genotype.

Digestion

Located in the stomach; secrete HCl and various enzymes (e.g. pepsin) when stimulated by gastrin.

PHENOTYPE

Biology

Biology

HEPATIC PORTAL VEIN

Genetics

The percentage of people in a population with a certain genotype who express the associated phenotype.

Digestion

Carries nutrients (monosaccharides, amino acids, and small fatty acids) absorbed in the small intestine to the liver, where they are modified to enter circulation.

PENETRANCE

Biology

Biology

INTESTINAL GLANDS

Genetics

The failure of homologous chromosomes or sister chromatids to separate properly during meiosis I and meiosis II, respectively. This usually results in gametes that lack certain genes or have multiple copies of those genes.

Digestion

Secretes maltase, sucrase, lactase, aminopeptidase, dipeptidase, and enterokinase into the small intestine.

NONDISJUNCTION

Biology

Biology

LARGE INTESTINE

Genetics

A cross between two organisms where only one trait is being studied.

Digestion

Section of the GI tract that consists of the cecum, the colon, and the rectum. The major function of the large intestine is to absorb salts and water.

MONOHYBRID CROSS

Biology

Biology

MECHANICAL DIGESTION

Genetics

Mendel's postulation that there are alternate versions of genes that account for genetic variation. Each individual has two alleles for each gene: one maternal and one paternal in origin. During meiosis, these two alleles separate into two different gametes.

Digestion

Breakdown of food particles into smaller particles through such activities as biting, chewing, and churning.

MENDEL'S LAW OF SEGREGATION

Biology

Genetics

The alleles of different genes assort independently during meiosis. We now know that this is only true for unlinked genes.

PANCRE

Digestion

Secretes pancreatic amylase, trypsin, chymotrypsin, carboxypeptidase, and lipase into the small intestine.

MENDEL'S LAW OF INDEPENDENT ASSORTMENT

Biology

Biology

PERISTALSIS

Genetics

Genes that are located on the same chromosome.

Digestion

Involuntary muscular contractions of the esophagus that push food down the digestive tract.

LINKED GENES

Biology

Biology

PYLORIC GLANDS

Genetics

A form of chromosomal rearrangement in which a portion of a chromosome breaks off and rejoins the same chromosome in the reverse position.

Digestion

Glands located in the walls of the stomach that secrete the hormone gastrin in response to certain substances in food.

INVERSION

Biology

Biology

PYLORIC SPHINCTER

Genetics

Describes a situation in which an organism heterozygous for a trait will have a phenotype that is intermediate to both alleles. Neither allele, therefore, is dominant or recessive.

Digestion

A valve between the stomach and the small intestine that regulates the flow of chyme into the small intestine.

INCOMPLETE DOMINANCE

Biology

Biology

SMALL INTESTINE

Genetics

Organisms that contain two identical copies of the same gene on corresponding chromosomes.

Digestion

The small intestine can be subdivided into three sections: the duodenum, jejunum, and the ileum. Most digestion takes place in the duodenum and most absorption takes place in the jejunum and the ileum.

HOMOZYGOUS

Biology

Biology

VILLI

Genetics

Organisms that contain two different alleles for the same gene on corresponding chromosomes.

Digestion

Fingerlike projections that extend out of the small intestine in order to increase surface area for maximum absorption.

HETEROZYGOUS

Biology

Biology

EXPIRATORY RESERVE VOLUME

Genetics

The genetic makeup of an individual.

Respiration

The amount of air that can be forcibly exhaled after a normal exhalation.

GENOTYPE

Biology

Biology

HYPERVENTILATION

Genetics

The degree to which an organism expresses its genotype.

Respiration

An increase in the rate of inhalation. Lack of oxygen or an increase in blood pH promotes hyperventilation.

EXPRESSIVITY

Biology

Biology

INTRAPLEURAL SPACE

A cross between two organisms where two distinct traits are being studied.

Genetics

Respiration

The space between the two membranes (visceral pleura and parietal pleura) that cover the lungs.

DIHYBRID CROSS

Biology

Biology

NEGATIVE PRESSURE BREATHING

Nervous System

Ends of axons that form one side of the synaptic cleft and where neurotransmitters are stored.

Respiration

The contraction of the diaphragm and the intercostal muscles increases the volume of the thoracic cavity, reducing the pressure in the intrapleural space. This decrease in pressure creates a vacuum which causes the lungs to suck in air.

SYNAPTIC TERMINALS

Biology

PASSAGE OF AIR DURING INHALATION

Nervous System

The space between the axon terminal of one neuron and the dendrite of another neuron where neurotransmitters are released.

Respiration

Air travels through the pharynx, larynx, trachea, bronchi, bronchioles, and then finally alveoli (site of gas exchange).

Biology

RESIDUAL VOLUME

Nervous System

Division of the peripheral nervous system that is responsible for voluntary movement.

Respiration

The amount of air that must remain in the lung at all times in order to prevent lung collapse.

SOMATIC NERVOUS SYSTEM

Biology

Biology

SURFACTANT

Nervous System

The white covering of the eye. Made up of connective tissue.

Respiration

A liquid substance produced by the lung that reduces surface tension in the alveoli. Surfactant prevents lung collapse and decreases the effort needed to expand the lungs (inhale).

SCLERA

Biology

Biology

TIDAL VOLUME

Nervous System

Cells that produce myelin in the peripheral nervous system.

Respiration

The volume of air that is normally inhaled or exhaled with each breath.

SCHWANN CELLS

Biology

Biology

TOTAL LUNG CAPACITY

Nervous System

A means by which action potentials jump from node to node along an axon.

Respiration

The maximum volume of air that the lung can hold which includes the vital capacity and the residual volume.

SALTATORY CONDUCTION

Biology

Biology

VITAL CAPACITY

Nervous System

A thin layer of cells containing photoreceptors at the back of the eye that converts light signals into neural impulses.

Respiration

The maximum volume of air that can be inhaled or exhaled by the lungs with each breath.

RETINA

Biology

Biology

ACTIVE IMMUNITY

Nervous System

The charge difference (maintained by the Na^+/K^+ pump) across the cell membrane of a neuron or a muscle cell while at rest.

Circulation

Immunity resulting from the production of antibodies during a previous infection or a vaccination.

RESTING POTENTIAL

Biology

Biology

ARTERIES

Nervous System

A process that occurs when the voltage-gated Na^+ channels close and voltage-gated K^+ channels open, allowing K^+ to rush out of the cell and repolarize it.

Circulation

Vessels that carry blood away from the heart. These vessels are muscular and do not have valves.

REPOLARIZATION

Biology

Biology

ATRIA

Nervous System

Type of sensory receptor that monitors the body's position in space.

Circulation

The two thin-walled upper chambers of the heart. The right atrium receives deoxygenated blood from the vena cava while the left atrium receives oxygenated blood from the pulmonary vein.

PROPRIOCEPTORS

Biology

Biology

ATRIOVENTRICULAR VALVES

Light-sensitive proteins.

Nervous System

Circulation

Valves located between the atria and the ventricles (tricuspid valve and mitral valve).

PHOTORECEPTORS

Biology

Nervous System

All neurons that are not part of the central nervous system, including sensory and motor neurons that connect to the central nervous system. Can be divided into the somatic nervous system and the autonomic nervous system.

BLOOD ANTIGENS

Biology

Circulation

Proteins found on the erythrocyte cell-surface. Three antigens used to differentiate blood groups are A, B, and Rh. If a host organism is transfused with erythrocytes containing antigens that the host does not have, an immune response will be triggered, such as in the case of erythroblastosis fetalis.

PERIPHERAL NERVOUS SYSTEM

Biology

Biology

BOHR EFFECT

Nervous System

Gaps in between segments of myelin sheath where action potentials can take place. Allows for saltatory conduction.

Circulation

Increasing the concentration of H^+ and CO_2 reduces hemoglobin's affinity for oxygen allowing for the transfer of oxygen to cells that require it most.

NODES OF RANVIER

Biology

Biology

CAPILLARIES

Nervous System

Chemical messengers released from synaptic clefts of a neuron that can bind and stimulate a postsynaptic cell.

Circulation

Blood vessels composed of a single layer of endothelial cells facilitating exchange between the blood and interstitial fluid.

NEUROTRANSMITTERS

Biology

Biology

CARBONIC ANHYDRASE

Nervous System

A protein that hydrolyzes 1 ATP to transport 3 Na^+ out of the cell for every $2K^+$ it transports into the cell.

Circulation

Enzyme that catalyzes the conversion of carbonic acid to carbon dioxide and water as well as the formation of carbonic acid from carbon dioxide and water.

NA^+/K^+ PUMP

Biology

Biology

CARDIAC OUTPUT

Nervous System

Insulating substance that surrounds axons. Action potentials cannot take place in areas of the axon that are myelinated.

Circulation

The total volume of blood the left ventricle pumps into circulation per minute. The cardiac output can be increased by increasing either the heart rate or the stroke volume.

MYELIN SHEATH

Biology

Biology

CORONARY ARTERIES

Nervous System

Reflex pathway that only has one synapse between the sensory neuron and the motor neuron.
Ex: knee-jerk reflex

Circulation

Blood vessels that supply the heart with oxygenated blood.

MONOSYNAPTIC REFLEX

Biology

Biology

CORONARY VEINS

Nervous System

The part of the brain that controls such functions as breathing and heartbeat.

Circulation

Blood vessels that transport deoxygenated blood from the heart toward the right atrium.

MEDULLA OBLONGATA

Biology

Biology

DIASTOLE

Nervous System

Muscular tissue that controls the amount of light allowed in through the pupil.

Circulation

The stage of the heart cycle in which the heart muscle relaxes and collects blood into its four chambers.

IRIS

Biology

Biology

ERYTHROCYTES

Nervous System

Type of sensory receptor that monitors blood pressure, the partial pressure of CO_2 in the blood, and the pH of blood within the body.

Circulation

The oxygen-carrying component of blood (red blood cells). These anaerobic cells, which lack organelles, are packed with hemoglobin and have a characteristic biconcave, disklike shape that facilitates gas exchange and mobility within blood vessels.

INTEROCEPTORS

Biology

Biology

FIBRIN

Nervous System

A group of neural cell bodies in the peripheral nervous system.

Circulation

Protein responsible for blood clotting.

GANGLIA

Biology

Biology

HEMOGLOBIN

Nervous System

Type of sensory receptor that monitors external signals such as light, sound, and temperature.

Circulation

A protein found in erythrocytes made up of four polypeptide chains, each containing a heme group. Hemoglobin is responsible for transporting oxygen from the alveoli to the cells.

EXTEROCEPTORS

Biology

Biology

HUMORAL IMMUNITY

Nervous System

Neurons that carry information from the central nervous system to other parts of the body.

Circulation

The synthesis of specific antibodies by activated B-cells in response to an antigen. These antibodies bind the antigen and either clump together to become insoluble or attract other cells that engulf them.

EFFERENT NEURONS

Biology

Biology

IMMUNOGLOBULINS

Nervous System

A process that occurs when the voltage-gated Na^+ channels open, allowing Na^+ to rush into the cell and depolarize it.

Circulation

A protein antibody produced in response to a specific foreign substance that recognizes and binds to that specific antigen and triggers an immune response.

DEPOLARIZATION

Biology

Biology

INFERIOR VENA CAVA

Nervous System

An extension of the neuron that transmits impulses toward the cell body.

Circulation

A large vein that returns deoxygenated blood from the lower body and the extremities to the right atrium of the heart.

DENDRITES

Biology

LEUKOCYTES

Nervous System

The corpus callosum connects the left hemisphere with the right hemisphere and correlates their activities.

Circulation

(White blood cells) The component of blood involved in cell defense and immunity. Neutrophils, basophils, eosinophils, lymphocytes, and monocytes are types of leukocytes.

CORPUS CALLOSUM

Biology

Biology

LYMPH NODES

Nervous System

Transparent covering in front of the eye that refracts light and helps keep the eye in focus.

Circulation

Swellings along the lymph vessels where lymph is filtered by leukocytes to remove antigens.

CORNEA

Biology

Biology

LYMPHATIC SYSTEM

Muscular tissue attached to the lens used to control the lens's shape.

Nervous System

Circulation

A system of vessels and lymph nodes that collect interstitial fluid and return them to the circulatory system thereby maintaining a plasma protein and fluid balance. The lymphatic system is also involved in lipid absorption and lymphocyte production.

CILIARY MUSCLES

Biology

Biology

MITRAL VALVE

Nervous System

The central nervous system consists of the brain and the spinal cord.

Circulation

A valve located between the left atrium and the left ventricle. The valve consists of two cusps and prevents backflow of blood from the ventricles to the atria.

CENTRAL NERVOUS SYSTEM

Biology

Biology

PASSIVE IMMUNITY

Nervous System

The portion of the neuron that connects the cell body (soma) to the axon. The impulses the neuron receives from all the dendrites are summed up at the axon hillock to determine if an action potential will be initiated.

Circulation

A short-lived immunity resulting from the transfer of antibodies into an individual who does not produce those antibodies.

AXON HILLOCK

Biology

Biology

PATH OF ELECTRICAL IMPULSE

Nervous System

Neurons that carry information to the central nervous system.

Circulation

The electrical impulse originates in the sinoatrial (SA) node, located in the right atrium. It then travels through the atrioventricular (AV) node, followed by the bundle of His, and finally through the Purkinje fibers.

AFFERENT NEURONS

Biology

Biology

PORTAL SYSTEMS

Nervous System

A sharp change in the membrane potential of neurons or muscle cells caused by a change in the selective permeability to K^+ and Na^+ using ion-gated channels. Action potentials are all-or-none events.

Circulation

Circulatory routes in which blood travels through two capillary beds before returning to the heart. Some examples include the hepatic portal system, the renal portal system, and the hypophyseal portal system.

ACTION POTENTIAL

Biology

Endocrine System

Synthesized and released by the anterior pituitary, TSH stimulates the thyroid gland to absorb iodine so that it can synthesize and secrete thyroid hormome. TSH is regulated by thyroid-releasing hormone (TRH), which is released by the hypothalamus.

PRIMARY RESPONSE

Circulation

The initial response to a specific antigen. During a primary response, T and B lymphocytes are activated and specific antibodies and memory cells to the antigen are produced.

THYROID-STIMULATING HORMONE

Biology

Endocrine System

Synthesized and released by the thyroid gland, thyroid hormones (Thyroxine, T4, and Triiodothyronine) stimulate cellular respiration as well as protein and fatty acid synthesis and degradation.

SECONDARY RESPONSE

Biology

Circulation

Subsequent infections by antigens trigger a more immediate response by the memory cells produced during the primary response.

THYROID HORMONES

Biology

Endocrine System

Hormone secreted by the interstitial cells of the testes. Testosterone is responsible for embryonic sexual differentiation, male sexual development, and the maintenance of masculine secondary sexual characteristics.

SEMILUNAR VALVES

Biology

Circulation

Valves that prevent backflow of blood from the arteries back into the ventricles (aortic valve and pulmonic valve).

TESTOSTERONE

Biology

SUPERIOR VENA CAVA

Nonpolar hormones that permeate the cell membrane and act by binding intracellular receptors.

Circulation

A large vein that returns deoxygenated blood from the head and neck regions to the right atrium of the heart.

STEROID HORMONES

Biology

Biology

SYSTOLE

Endocrine System

Produced and secreted by the delta cells of the pancreas, somatostatin inhibits the release of glucagon and insulin.

Circulation

The stage of the heart cycle in which the heart muscle contracts and pumps blood.

SOMATOSTATIN

Biology

Biology

TRICUSPID VALVE

Endocrine System

A hormone synthesized and released by the anterior pituitary that stimulates milk production and secretion in female mammary glands.

Circulation

A valve located between the right atria and the right ventricle. The valve consists of three cusps and prevents backflow of blood from the ventricle to the atria.

PROLACTIN

Biology

Endocrine System

Hormone synthesized and released by the ovaries, corpus luteum, and placenta. During the luteal phase of the menstrual cycle, the corpus luteum secretes progesterone, which, along with estrogen, stimulates the development and maintenance of the endometrial walls for implantation of the embryo.

VEINS

Biology

Circulation

Vessels that carry blood toward the heart. These vessels are thin-walled and have valves to prevent backflow.

PROGESTERONE

Biology

Biology

VENTRICLES

Endocrine System

Stores and releases hormones (oyxtocin and ADH) synthesized by the hypothalamus. The release of these hormones is triggered by an action potential that originates in the hypothalamus.

Circulation

The muscular lower chambers of the heart. The right ventricle pumps deoxygenated blood to the lungs through the pulmonary artery while the left ventricle pumps oxygenated blood throughout the body.

POSTERIOR PITUITARY

Biology

Endocrine System

Polar hormones incapable of permeating the cell membrane that bind to surface receptors and act through secondary messengers.

Biology

ADH

Homeostasis

Antidiuretic hormone (ADH), also known as vasopressin, acts on the collecting duct to increase water reabsorption. ADH is produced by the hypothalamus and stored in the posterior pituitary.

PEPTIDE HORMONES

Biology

Endocrine System

Synthesized and released by the parathyroid gland, PTH increases blood Ca_2^+ concentration by increasing Ca_2^+ reabsorption in the kidneys and by stimulating calcium release from bone.

ALDOSTERONE

Biology

Homeostasis

A steroid hormone produced in the adrenal cortex responsible for reabsorption of sodium and water and the excretion of potassium.

PARATHYROID HORMONE

Biology

Biology

ASCENDING LIMB OF THE LOOP OF HENLE

Endocrine System

Synthesized and released by the anterior pituitary, LH stimulates ovulation and formation of the corpus luteum. LH is regulated by estrogen, progesterone, and gonadotropin-releasing hormone (GnRH).

Homeostasis

Portion of the nephron not permeable to water. As the filtrate flows up the ascending limb through decreasing concentration of the interstitial fluid, Na^+ is actively pumped out of the filtrate decreasing filtrate concentration.

LUTEINIZING HORMONE

Biology

COLLECTING DUCT

Endocrine System

Produced and secreted by the beta cells of the pancreas, insulin decreases blood glucose concentrations by facilitating the uptake of glucose by muscle and adipose cells and the conversion of glucose to glycogen in muscle and liver cells.

Homeostasis

Portion of the nephron permeable to water and ions. As the filtrate flows down the collecting duct through the increasing concentration of the interstitial fluid, the filtrate is concentrated further. The degree of water reabsorption in the collecting duct is controlled by the action of the hormones ADH and aldosterone.

INSULIN

Biology

Biology

DERMIS

Endocrine System

Synthesized and released by the anterior pituitary, GH stimulates bone and muscle growth as well as glucose conservation. GH is inhibited by somatostatin and stimulated by Growth Hormone–Releasing Hormone (secreted by the hypothalamus).

Homeostasis

The layer of skin beneath the epidermis that is subdivided into the papillary layer and the reticular layer. It contains the sweat glands, sense organs, blood vessels, and the bulbs of hair follicles, and is derived from the mesoderm.

GROWTH HORMONE

Biology

DESCENDING LIMB OF THE LOOP OF HENLE

Endocrine System

Synthesized and released by the adrenal cortex, glucocorticoids raise blood glucose levels while decreasing protein synthesis.

Homeostasis

Portion of the nephron only permeable to water. The filtrate becomes more concentrated (loses water) as it travels through the descending limb due to the increasing concentration of the interstitial fluid.

GLUCOCORTICOIDS

Biology

Endocrine System

Produced and secreted by the alpha cells of the pancreas, glucagon increases blood glucose concentration by promoting gluconeogenesis and the conversion of glycogen to glucose in the liver.

EPIDERMIS

Biology

Homeostasis

The outermost layer of skin composed of the following sublayers: stratum basalis, stratum spinosum, stratum granulosum, stratum lucidum, and stratum corneum. Serves as a protective barrier against microbial attack. Derived from the ectoderm.

GLUCAGON

Biology

Endocrine System

Synthesized and released by the anterior pituitary, FSH stimulates maturation of ovarian follicles in females and maturation of the seminiferous tubules and sperm production in males. FSH is regulated by estrogen and gonadotropin-releasing hormone (GnRH).

Biology

FILTRATE

Homeostasis

The material that passes from the blood vessels into Bowman's capsule.

FOLLICLE-STIMULATING HORMONE

Biology

Endocrine System

Glands that synthesize and secrete substances through ducts. The gall bladder is an example of an exocrine gland.

GLOMERULUS

Biology

Homeostasis

Network of capillaries within Bowman's capsule that serves as the site of filtration. Blood cells and proteins are too large to be filtered but ions, glucose, and amino acids readily pass into the filtrate.

EXOCRINE GLANDS

Biology

Biology

GLUCONEOGENESIS

Endocrine System

Hormone synthesized and released by the ovaries, the ovarian follicles, the corpus luteum, and the placenta. Estrogen stimulates the development of the female reproductive tract and secondary sexual characteristics and is partly responsible for the LH spike that causes ovulation. Estrogen, along with progesterone produced by the placenta during the second trimester of pregnancy, helps inhibit the onset of a new menstrual cycle by blocking GnRH release.

Homeostasis

A process in the liver by which glucose is produced using by-products of glycolysis, lipids, or fats.

ESTROGEN

Biology

Biology

HYPODERMIS

Endocrine System

Synthesized and released by the anterior pituitary, endorphins inhibit the perception of pain.

Homeostasis

Layer of loose connective tissue below the dermis that binds the dermis to the body.

ENDORPHINS

Biology

Biology

NEPHRON

Endocrine System

Glands that synthesize and secrete hormones into the circulatory system. Examples include the hypothalamus, pituitary gland, pineal gland, thymus, pancreas, testes, ovaries, adrenal glands, thyroid gland, and parathyroid glands.

Homeostasis

The functional unit of the kidney. Can be subdivided into Bowman's capsule, proximal convoluted tubule, descending limb of the loop of Henle, ascending limb of the loop of Henle, distal convoluted tubule, and the collecting duct.

ENDOCRINE GLANDS

Biology

Biology

OSMOREGULATION

Endocrine System

Tissue that forms from the collapsed ovarian follicle. Produces and secretes progesterone and estrogen.

Homeostasis

Maintenance of water and solute concentrations.

CORPUS LUTEUM

Biology

PROXIMAL CONVOLUTED TUBULE

Endocrine System

Hormone synthesized and released by the thyroid gland that decreases plasma $Ca_{2}{}^{+}$ concentration.

Homeostasis

Site where glucose, amino acids, and other important organic molecules are reabsorbed. The proximal convoluted tubules lie in the cortex of the kidney.

CALCITONIN

Biology

Endocrine System

Synthesizes and releases many vital hormones including follicle-stimulating hormone, luteinizing hormone, adrenocorticotropic hormone, thyroid-stimulating hormone, prolactin, endorphins, and growth hormone ("FLAT PEG"). The anterior pituitary is under the hormonal control of the hypothalamus.

THERMOREGULATION

Biology

Homeostasis

Maintenance of a constant internal body temperature.

ANTERIOR PITUITARY

Biology

ADRENAL CORTEX

Endocrine System

Hormones that are synthesized from amino acids. Some amino acid derived hormones act via secondary messengers while others act in a similar fashion to steroid hormones.

Endocrine System

Synthesizes and releases corticosteroids (including glucocorticoids and mineralcorticoids) when stimulated by adrenocorticotropic hormone (ACTH).

AMINO ACID DERIVED HORMONES

Biology

Endocrine System

Synthesized and released by the anterior pituitary, ACTH stimulates the adrenal cortex to synthesize and secrete glucocorticoids. ACTH is regulated by corticotrophin-releasing hormone (CRF), which is released by the hypothalamus.

ADRENAL MEDULLA

Biology

Endocrine System

Synthesizes and releases epinephrine and norepinephrine, which stimulate an increase in the metabolic rate and blood glucose levels.

ADRENOCORTICOTROPIC HORMONE

Biology

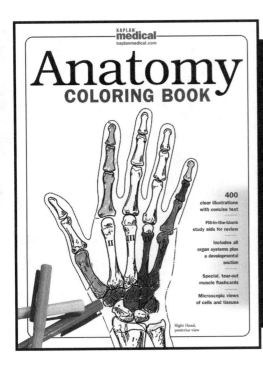